Like A Fi of C

CW00833177

John Ryan

chipmunkapublishing

the mental health publisher

John Ryan

Published by

Chipmunkapublishing

PO Box 6872

Brentwood

Essex CM13 1ZT

United Kingdom

http://www.chipmunkapublishing.com

Chipmunkapublishing gratefully acknowledge the sup-port of Arts Council England.

Author Biography

Six years ago, one day changed John Ryan's life for ever. Just another day at work, it seemed, until he was approached from behind by a much younger man, who buggered him with such force that John suffered a complete mental breakdown, which has lasted to this day.

This volume of poems is a detailed description of the journey of that breakdown.

John, now 63, is determined to recover that he hopes to begin a Degree at University in September 2010, reading Anthropology and Sociology. This volume is dedicated to those who suffered with him during his three-time stay in a mental institution.

John Ryan

# Like A Fine Piece of China

A Mental Institution

Gates chained, doors locked, freedom lost,
language at a minimum, grunts and groans
the extent of my loquacity: silent responses,
shock after shock, learning to queue, 'they
also serve who only stand and wait'. Strange
bed, stranger dreams. Glassy-eyed stares,
no words wasted, the shock of dislodgement.
Assessments yet again, here in formal mode,
no chance of release for a month or more, yet
no crime admitted. Counting each minute of
each hour of each day of each week. Enough
to drive one to the verge. Staring out my
window, I follow the bird's free movement
with mounting anger and hopelessness. Why
has it come to this? "A danger to oneself and
to others". I laugh stoically. Dead leaves fall
this autumn,: were they, in their green glory,
ever as radiant as this, in death? I hear the
hum of the busy world beyond, my proper
world - this world I will have no assent to,
but cope I must, and will.

ABUSED

Being used and abused made my soul dark
to the point of infinite pain;
I lost all my mind and all of my soul
it's a wonder I'm still fully sane.

I've been down to the depths of a bottomless pit
- the pain was unbearable then;
as I look back on my previous life
I am shocked and surprised as to when

I suffered a massive mental breakdown
which I would not wish on another;
but I have pulled through and am now quite sane
because we did all this together.

Excruciating pain is a terrible thing
it caused me to scream and to cry,
but now I'm on the mend with a very close friend
my eyes are now fully dry.

I'm still locked away in my room all day
- all night if the truth be told,
for I am scared to go out in the street
I am not yet that forward or bold.

Adult abuse is a wicked crime
as is child abuse in my books,
but there are people out there who pray to their gods
yet in private they are nothing but crooks.

Abuse is abuse, it has to be said,
abuse is a crime still today:
in spite of the fact that people forget
and go to their churches to pray.

Like A Fine Piece of China

I'm so angry at what to me was then done,
was depressed and I wanted to die;
suicide then seemed an option quite clear,
but now I will settle to cry.

Why I allowed the abuse so to be
is a mystery beyond my mind;
I should have had it stopped right there and then
yet I think that you will somehow find

That good folk are scared when they are abused
- scared of what might happen right now;
if they should ever tell and have it be known
that they are involved in a row.

My pain was intense as I was abused
I laid on my bed just to cry;
Now I'm recovering, I do want to know
an answer to the question "Why?"

My heart does go out to all who're like me,
they suffered in silence, too;
no more will I suffer, for I'm on the mend
- like me, there are simply too few.

If you've been like me, abused in the dark
I urge you to stand real tall:
let's stand together against the abuse
and never again let us stall.

After Intense Pain

After intense pain
comes a feeling
of numbness, a
lesser pain that is
almost bearable.
Nature looks
for a balance,
after extremes
of pain. Which is
why I am, today,
at a kind of
temporary
ceasefire
after the
intensity of
recent pain . . .

ALONE

Too many times I've sat alone,
sat there and not answered the phone,
and all because I am prone
to stay all day on my own.

I have suffered a lot in my time
and yet I've committed no crime;
I'm here on my bed just lying
depressed, and I've just started crying.

My psychiatrist says I'm delusional
- which isn't all that unusual
if you consider the circumstances for me
- used to be happy, but now I'm not free

to be my old self anymore
but now I do set great store
on this man's advice, to me he's so nice
and I trust him and all his advice.

Delusions are such a curse,
but I suffer from conditions much worse
I pray that I'll keep all my health
- much more important than wealth.

I'll be back to old me pretty soon
I shall sing my old songs (and in tune!)
- barring relapses that are bad,
and I shall no longer be sad.

ALONE (2)

All alone, yet full of mental strength
To face the daily grind together with
My poems so uplifting in my soul.
The world says No, don't be alone,
But I say Be alone, and search the
Meaning further still. My days ain't
Long enough for projects such as this,
Such is my delight dissembling words
And words and words.

All alone this hour, masticating in my
Lair, giving birth to new-laid forms of
Words that stimulate the appetite for
More, facing up to long-held
Mysteries - hoping that I might be
A newly-minted Me.

ALONE AGAIN

And I am alone again, creating silence
as an aid to concentration, entering
deep into a conversation with myself.
For I hardly know myself, and others
even less.

Yet, I know silence intimately, for it is
a state of being. Alone: frowned upon,
but full of creativity. Silence is my
closest friend; serving our mutual
needs we create delightful duets.

And so I'm not alone again.

Among Friends

I've been up all night and now I'm tired,
it's early morning but I am fired
with energy from all at this site
they've helped to make my load so light.

The reassurance is helpful indeed,
it's helped me in my hour of need;
I'll be coming back again and again
it's taken away so much of the strain.

Thank you all for so much strength,
now I've got courage for so much of the length
of the road ahead, and it's due to you,
thank you one and all: this is so true.

ANGER

Anger that is suppressed is anger not at all:
this is how I have been angry all this long,
long time. Peaceful folk want lives of peace
- anger seems unnatural. But come this
righteous anger fully clothed in battle-dress
and life is changed fore'er.

Suppressing anger is the road to hell.
Unable to express it, let me tell,
is fatal; now I know just what to do –
this is my tale: it could be you.
"Don't keep it all inside" they said
but me? I kept it all inside, to bed
I went with anger in my head.

The time had come to check my health
for I recognised not all the wealth
could compensate, were I to suppress by stealth
the smothering anger any more. Then I stepped
alone but with determination, slowly crept
to a safer, silent world of inner peace,
a peace that was a newer lease
of life, for suppression brought a world of pain
that made me sick, no longer sane.

It was then I realised that suppression made
for doom, and in my bed for days I laid
in torment; but now upon my bed I sleep
in peace, I pray my guardian angel keep
me so. My days of brutal pain are o'er:
my inner soul no longer tore
to shreds, for the lesson I've to tell
is simple: avoid the road to hell
by opening up to anger well.

John Ryan

AT THE END

When all the times have come to nought,
And all life's battles were well fought:
Who is to say what might be, now,
Remembering the high and low

Of life's long way, viewed in a blink,
The way it is, or so I think;
That long road's coming to the end,
Life's lovely garden I did tend

With diligence, and loving care,
That garden's brimming – 'twas once bare;
And I am ready to depart,
And from that road I will depart.

And who's to say what will be then,
I do so wish this I could pen
For everyone and all to see
- On this road I've been true to ME.

AWAKE!

Awake! 'tis time to be awake
And up, and busy with my verse,
For now the dawn has passed
And elves and fairies have retreated fast;
The sun is up, the day has come,
No more the dark enveloping around,
- Replaced by brilliant sunshine this happy
Summer morn'. And I can sense the Muse
This hour, flitting through the ether past
And willing to dispense her gifts to me
This time of plenty in the summer time.

Come! come! 'tis time to meditate
And ruminate and speak with gods
Of eloquence and share their wisdom
In my garden of delights.

The sun's already burning bright, the dew
On roses, beady-like, and all of Nature
Wide awake while mortals still do snore,
And only I am blissfully aware of Nature's wiles
This happy hour before the day begins anew.

BREAKDOWN

I used to be "normal" but now I'm so weak,
I take time as it comes, I live week by week.
My breakdown it came just out of the blue
I'm sad it is me but I'm glad it's not you.

God's in His heaven, the devil's in hell,
this is my story which I want to tell.
I was abused by a man determined to fight
to achieve his objective: sexual delight.

He achieved what he wanted - he was stronger than me,
he had his vile pleasure and so now you see
why I suffered a breakdown which lasts to this day;
I suffer intensely - that's all I can say.

But I am amazed at the good folk I've met
who told me they love me and that I shouldn't fret.
But you see, I don't know if I can trust anyone:
I live in the darkness away from the sun.

I really do want to trust humankind,
but my trust has been shattered and so has my mind.
I suffer depression as black as can be;
I suffer paranoia - that is the new me.

My memory's gone, I have blackouts as well,
but it gives me release this story to tell.
It's very good therapy to write down my life,
I wish it were happier instead of this strife.

Think kindly, dear reader, of someone like me
who's sitting and staring while under the tree.

Sitting and staring for hours at an end,
for I look for some comfort from you, my dear friend.

Some people can suffer, and still can endure
the most awful privations - they are saints to be sure.
I'm no saint, nor an angel - I am simply just me,
that's why I do suffer, while under that tree.

My memory's gone, my mind is too weak
to bear all this pain, and so I do seek
release from this cross, release from the pain,
I pray to high heaven that I will stay sane.

I'm angry and bitter, yet forgiving and good;
I'm mixed in my emotions, but I know that I should
forgive all the trauma, the hurt and the pain
- I have to do this if I want to remain sane.

I am scared to go out, I am scared of all men,
as I sit in my room which is now just a den;
this is my prison, as I look for the moon
through a long night of suffering which I hope will end
soon.

My psychiatrist he thinks he can fix my mind,
there is every good chance, as he's gentle and kind;
If I could get back to where I used to be
I would be so happy, for I would be free.

Thank you, kind reader, for hearing my tale,
I'm still feeling sad, because I'm quite frail;
but I feel so much better for telling it through,
May the good Lord in heaven look after you.

Bullying

Day by day, drip by drip,
incessantly, how it began
to register on the mind, the
clammy, sweaty fear, fear
of the bully, of folk in general,
even doubting my own judgement:
undermined.
Why me? I asked myself. I was
polite, gentle and truthful to the
last. Now it's all over, but I lost
my job and then my mind . . .
I'm still polite, gentle and truthful
to the last . . .then the nightmares,
the twitching of the feet as I fall off
to sleep.
Incessant bullying, so insidious, so
damned unjust, the bully with his
smug respectability, a pillar of moral
rectitude, but rotten to the core, I
pray the gods he'll get his
comeuppance. . .
Forgive, they say, forgive, but so far
I can't forgive. I certainly can't forget.
May the gods forgive me for a change,
forgive my anger,
my boiling anger . . .

Composing

Pacing up and down,
nervously picking my nose,
scratching, needing to get
my inner voice in order,
the agony of indecision,
scared to mark my virgin
page lest a plodding mind
betray a vacuous mind
this early morning hour.

The pain of indecision, the
wavering process on a cold
mind, utterly devoid of a
spark to free that mind once
more. Originality vomits
crude notions upon the
 empty page - tempted to
let it be: for the sake of
scratches here and there.

So much easier to wallow
in a fool's distraction, yet
who can tell if fools don't
make some sense?

Darkness

Dark is my mind with pain,
my soul with depression.
Night covers all with her
cloak, so dark I cannot
negotiate the back-alleys
of my own mind.
I am brooding alone,
but no self-pity. Simply
enduring. Sitting endlessly,
twiddling my thumbs,
studying the moon. Numb
to my core, I am not
sufficiently numb to escape
intense mental pain.
The years'-long winter has
finally struck home. The
howling Voices have worn
my soul bare. Fair-weather
friends have camped in the
sunlit lowlands. Years
of endurance have left their
mark, such that now I am at
a kind of inner peace. Worse
than a toothache, the mental
pain is gnawing at my very
soul. The mental pain cannot
be extracted, though I have
been 'treated' endlessly by
clinicians. The midday sun is
on another planet. All my mind
experiences is eternal darkness.
Pockets of optimism are, like
shooting stars, momentary.

The return of daylight to my
mind is imperceptible, if at all.
But it comes. Yet, even the
hazy midday sun is too low to
thaw that tired, tired mind. All
too soon, the short day is o'er.

DEPRESSION

Depression, my old friend, rings my bell
and asks for tea. The world is open for
business as usual – but I'm not buying.

I steal an hour of counselling but wish
the hell the label fell from round my
neck. No such luck. I'm home alone,
surrounded by the city noise, depression
is my one true friend. We share, why,
we even sleep together: inseparable.

"Give her up" they plead – "go shopping
- good therapy" But I'm not buying. Not
now, not ever. It's one a.m. The door-bell
rings, I can't resist, yet I hate this affair.
I once held Sleep captive at this hour, put
a notice up LOST: BEAUTIFUL SLEEP, and
how I grieve the loss.

Depression wants to caress me, smother
me; yet I'm moulded into its ways and
idiosyncrasies, utterly captivated. I truly
hate the complicity. Caught between
fascination and exhaustion. We have tea
again. The dark outside is a metaphor for
my soul. If only I could cry: no such luck.
Depression overstays the welcome, but
I'm mesmerized, unable to escape.

The early sun filters through my soul,
another wasted night, I wallow in
despair as, imperceptibly, depression
makes a run for it.

DREAMS

Why do dreams upset me so?
for dreams can be a source
of joy supreme – but not for me.
I look for respite in the night
- all I get is pain and fright,
a repetition of the scary stuff
that makes me plead "I've had enough"
"Why now?", I plead – "Why me?"
"just go away and give me peace"
for night is time for rest and sleep,
my angel in its bosom keep.

But no – for me the demons come
to have their pleasure out of sun,
they play by moonlight in the dark
and when I wake they've left their mark
on a soul too tired to scream "Away!"
and yet "Away!" I manage to say
as early birds the morrow greet
exhaustion is my morning treat.

Farewell the pleasures of the moon,
a new day dawns , so now quite soon
I'll recount my dreams including screams
that only demons know and share;
for I'm too tired, my soul lies bare
the sun is up, maybe to share
the certainty of daylight: that's all I care,
the heat of sun upon my face
and demons of the night no trace
may leave, instead the sun's rays on my face.

Dusk to Night

Hail! The dusk,
precursor of the night,
great is my joy,
my anticipation
of pleasures to come.

Night, the time of silence
and fulsome pleasures
of the mind;
great is my joy.

The mind at its most creative,
the soul, its most solemn,
the spirit, its most vigorous,
the conscience, its cleanest,
great is my joy.

Hail! The hours of moon-lit joy,
holy orb transmitting vibes
to sentient soul, awake,
alive to what it has to offer
- great is my joy.

Early Morning

I open my eyes and I hear cries in my heart
- I was awake all night, my soul is a clutter
as I hear myself mutter expletives best not
repeated in polite company.

Insomnia is a close friend, but selfish and
demanding on every point. Paranoia is not
far behind, demanding to be attended to,
even at night. Like a baby, he must be fed.

I'm moody, grumpy, irritable: not nice to
know first thing. Yet it's contradictory, I
want so much to love, to be pleasant. I'm
getting such a raw deal from life's lottery.

I went to bed in the blackest mood – to
bed, but not to sleep. I did all the wrong
things: I smoked, I cried, I railed against
the gods. And all because of my other

close friend, deep, deep chronic Depression.
There's one saving grace: I'm chirpy at this
ungodly early hour, wide awake. I get a kind
of 'second breath'. Instinct and experience

drive me to my writing. I stare at the blank
screen, get writer's block, and cry – again.
Does anyone understand my isolation, can
anyone empathise, share my plight for even

a passing second, I ask myself. Dull, dozing
Depression will not budge, so why do I keep
such company? The psychiatrist has diagnosed

me with a raft of conditions, but why

Depression? Up all night, not even tired, can
someone explain? I don't go out – at all – so
I shall be my own exclusive company all day.
But with one difference: Light has come.

The others are livid at her arrival: jealous. But
Light doesn't talk, she operates in secret, and
there's the problem: I talk to myself. All day
and all night. I've pleaded with these guys to

leave, and so often, but no one's budging. I'm
half-resigned to my fate. My face is showing
my age, my lack of sleep, my battle with
Depression. I don't apologise anymore for my

choice of company. Now I'm suddenly dopey,
Sleep, a relative stranger, casts her spell on me
and who knows, she may cast a spell on these
others. Her spell is potent, I'm finished with this.

FOR ALL THE TIMES

For all the times when times were good,
A little of Life is understood;
For all the times when times were bad,
A lot of Life was so, so sad.

But optimistic moods are near
And help to stop the dreaded tear;
And Life defeats all comers still,
And drops sweet music in the till.

Oh yes, if we could but enjoy
Each moment as it passes by:
Our lives would be so much enriched
And misery would then be ditched.

Ye gods, that we may walk around
Life's pleasure garden newly found,
And find the strength to face the day,
And throw the negatives away.

Life, after all, is e'er so rich
If only we could throw the stitch
That binds the goodness and the bad,
- Begone the bits that make us sad.

For we must optimistic be
And travel far from sea to sea,
And in that process happy be,
For that is Life's sure legacy.

Full Moon

I welcome the night
without a fight,
I welcome the morn
a new day is born,
I welcome the sun,
the old night is done.
I'm awake through the night
I hang in there tight,
I peer at the moon:
it'll be gone all too soon,
the full moon is my peer
and it holds no fear
for me, now or never,
I don't want to sever
my enjoyment as I look
at its grace, it's a book.
Its chapters do send
notes to a friend
through the night hours
- the night is all ours.
Adieu the full moon
yes it's gone all too soon
I welcome the sun,
the old night is done.

Gentle and Kind

I'm old and kind
but of unsound mind,
I suffer from depression
because of repression;
I kept it all inside
in my soul and in my mind.
My friend take heed,
and watch my deed,
follow my advice
- be gentle and nice.
We all need each other
sister and brother
though of unsound mind
I'm gentle and kind
I've leant a lot through my long life at home
It pays to be kind though I no longer roam,
It pays to be gentle, though my face be lined
through life's worries, I look after my mind.
My depression is lifting already today
the sun it is shining, I think I'll make hay
I feel better for writing, this is off my chest
be gentle and kind, and be my guest.

Good Moods and Bad

Yesterday I was up
today I'm down,
yesterday I was smiling,
Today I've a frown.
That is how my condition is,
that's how it goes, you see,
but I'm slowly improving day by day
- that's how I want it to be.
It's a difficult life being just like this,
a life full of turmoil and pain,
I'm on my tablets every day
 - that way, I hope to remain sane.

Healing at Last

I am healing at last,
slowly sleeping off the pain,
slowly ridding myself of the
psychological scars; slowly
ridding myself of the numbness
which accompanies trauma
and depression.
My pain is deep, and I'm weak,
so the movements of my mind
are cumbersome. I see folk out
of my window rushing to work,
I, too, work on my recuperation,
alone. Always alone.
Officials see me regularly, good
folk they are, but have they, I
ask myself, been to my hell? I
think not. You don't come out
of my hell, merely learn to cope.
My healing is merely my coping,
but there is no escape. That is
why I will never get back to my
old self. But do I want to? We
have to move-on to someone
new. Bury the old. That was
then, this is now. My healing
will make me a new me. The
pain of transference, the pain
of growth, the pain of becoming
a new me.
There will be relapses, but an
unstoppable movement to a new
growth, sending out new shoots.
Nature in the raw, working

incessantly to survive: to survive
the hell I've inhabited all these
years. Strange being out and
about, within the strict confines
of my home, as going outside
is simply not an option.
Scared of the world, getting
out there will come in slow,
deliberate steps. I don't want
that world, I want my own
company exclusively. That is a
measure of my condition. A lot
of healing ahead, for sure.

I Love You

The wise man said: "Sensibility, not knowledge,
is what is needed".
These words I've pondered and now I've heeded.
The early sun has brought the light,
but when I look at you I get a fright;
you are not the one you used to be,
you're in your black hole for, it seems, eternity.
Your depression is making you feel so blue,
I love you so much, for you are you.
I want you out from your deep, black hole,
I want you to be happy in body and soul,
this will happen in its own good time,
you are so innocent, you've done no crime;
look in my eyes and see the real me,
my love is exclusively only for thee.
If ever I find out that you might fail,
against the gods I will mightily rail,
why don't you go to your bed and lie,
if I ever did lose you, I would only want to die;
in the olden days you were always bright,
now you are a pitiful sight;
if I ever were able to tell my tale
we would be in a boat and we would sail
to the top of the world, then to the sky,
- this is a fantasy, for seeing you I cry,
you sleep in your bed, but your mood is low,
I never, ever dreamt that it would be so.
Don't be depressed, that is all I say
I love you, my darling, as on your bed you lay,
knowing your depression, fills me with fear,
I cherish you so much as I shed a tear.
I want you to be happy under the sky
but your moods are so low instead of being high;

Like A Fine Piece of China

it was always such pleasure with you to lie
but now this condition makes me want to die,
so now my dear precious as you still lay,
I love you, I love you: that's all I want to say.

I Walk Alone

The old city walls are crumbling to dust
as I take a lone walk, for walk I must
I walk alone, for I don't like a crowd,
- crowds are too noisy, and far, far too loud.
I've suffered mental illness for many a year
to the point that now I can only shed a tear,
the dust of the walls is like deep in my soul
- dry and uncomforted, life has taken its toll.
As I touch the dry walls and feel the very stones
of history in my hands, I hear the moans
of souls long dead, I hear the groans
of long-dead bodies, crumbling
like the walls, I hear wails of grumbling
at the manner of their death
- life owes them a terrible debt.
The traffic is honking, the people are noisy
and I am alone with my thoughts, alone
with these souls of yesteryear, I atone
in my soul for the gruesome way
they died, now I want to stay
and touch the dust, for souls now long gone,
brave souls upon whom the sun shone
but no more. I linger a moment,
and pray a prayer of atonement
for the dead and the quick
as I crumble yet another brick
in my dry hands, reflecting as I leave
on my simple faith, I believe.

I'M JUST ME

I'm just me
with all my faults
but in the psychiatric ward
they want me to be
someone else,
more "normal".

Dammit, I'm ME,
not an actor.
Be this, be that,
can I just
be ME?

I don't want to dress-up
I want to wear my own
mental clothes.

I want to be just me
I want to cry.
That's just being me.

 I'm confused:
"Be yourself -
but don't cry"
Don't do this
don't do that . . .

I want to be me
- I want a hug.
they don't do crying,
they don't do hugs.

Damn the lot of them:
I'm going to stay

as I am;
I'm going to be ME

I'M THINKING NOW

I'm thinking now of all the times
When I was young and wrote my rhymes
And everything was happy, bright,
- But it was all to end in fright,

For Life has taught me lessons hard,
Not easy being a wise old bard;
I'm older now and Life is slow,
There's little else I need to know.

Don't get me wrong – I'm happy still,
But happiness is tempered till
We reach a point in Life's hard way
- It's easy then, to go astray.

To go astray, avoiding pain,
Following the moon's slow wane,
Mistaking fortune for bad ilk,
Mistaking sherry for sour milk.

The human mind is frail and weak:
Composed of cardboard, not of teak;
I need those nerves of steel today -
Lest I Life's secrets do betray.

Indoors

I stay indoors by day
I stay indoors at night
I venture out not anytime
- it's too much of a fright.
That's the way I am today
the way it's been sometime,
the way I'll be tomorrow
- the way since I lost my prime.
Good were the days when I was me,
those were the days of peace,
before my troubles came along:
I wish that this would cease.
Mental health is a difficult one
to conquer and put right,
it takes all my time and energy
Lord, help me in my plight.
Many folk are the same as me
they suffer so much pain
they endure extreme agonies
in an effort to be sane.
Why we suffer I don't know,
why the pain? I ask
Lord give us the strength to cope
as we plod on with our task.
The fright it comes as I go out
to face the world again:
it doesn't clear as on I walk,
so I return home again.
That is where I am today
that is where I'll be
for that is who I am these days
for that is simply me.
I endure my pain with fortitude

Like A Fine Piece of China

with patience I survive,
for I am still a fighter
- I want to be alive.
I want to warm in the morning sun,
and have it in my face,
I want to enjoy the moon at night
its magic to embrace.
I don't intend to give-up the fight
I intend to soldier on,
my intention is to walk upright
- the wreath of success I'll don.

Insanity

The curse of instability:
hanging on to sanity,
the pain of concentration,
yesterday's breakdown
today's fragility, numbness.
Tense, tired, but sleep
evades.

From intensely private pain
to formalised white-coated
insanity, sanitised
officialdom.

"Come", they said, "we will
 save your pain" – but
do they know the pain?
Can they define the sane?

I can. I can define myself,
not insane, but in pain.

The new-born twig, so
full of potential,
struck down by a too-early
frost, me struck down
by a too-late insanity,
the frosty pain, the pain.

The frost evaporates
imperceptibly,
the pain grows more
intense, the pain.
No light in this soul,
the frosty pain, the pain.

INSOMNIA

I ruminate in my lair as I say a small prayer
while in the darkness everyone is snoring.
Night has cast her spell over the world, but I
am wide awake: listening to my Voice,
petrified to enter that world, night or day.
My bedroom is my castle. I sit by my window,
studiously engaged with the nocturnal predations
of Sister Moon, summoning up the courage to
face down my Voice should it scream at me again.

My hands are clammy and shaking as I roll another
fag. The pleasure my sexual attacker got, left me in
this state, now I cannot get him out of my mind: he
follows me to this day, or night, both mentally and
emotionally. Each night, I have flashbacks, all too
vivid. But it's the Voice that has climbed the turret
and bawls out to me suddenly – I jump momentarily,
startled. The advice is: "Acknowledge, negotiate, talk
back to the Voice". Words, words, words: if only I could.

I'm up most of the night, every night, Sleep's magic
passing me by. I creep around not wanting to wake
anyone. I write incessantly, have endless cups of tea,
and in fear of the Voice, I smoke too much. I am me,
dammit . . . I'm saturated with contradictory feelings:
anger, forgiveness, refusal to forgive, and jump invol-
untarily at the slightest sound. I'm not leaving my
castle. They can lay waste to the surrounding city: I'm
refusing to budge – its much too dangerous out there
where humankind wanders day and night. I'm pet-
rified of what's out there. Condemned as being
paranoid, I say I'm just being realistically cautious. Who
can blame me after what I've been through? Leave
me to be ME, I say . . . I enjoy my chosen methodolo-

gies,
after a fashion.

Two cats are fighting outside, and I can see the foxes
scavenging. I eke out my own existence, paltry as it is.
But I never force myself to sleep. Insomnia is my
friend, not a blasted curse. "Adaptability, old boy,
adaptability". I wish my attacker, my sexual predator,
could have adapted himself to the mores of civil
society. I wouldn't now be in the state I am. The cats
really are having a bitter fued.

They can give me all the medication they want, but I still
won't sleep. As I fill-up my tablet box for the next week,
the first bird begins twittering outside. Light is beckon-
ing,
it's been a long night, I can't bring myself to read, but do
spend a considerable time on the net. What would I do
without my computer? I'm getting dopey, but won't sleep

Last Night

My soul is yearning for the light of day
there are a number of things I want to say,
last night was a bad one (if I may say to you)
cold feet, bad dreams, other symptoms, too,
insomnia is awful, it cuts to the bone,
my soul it is leaden, heavy as a stone
depressed my heart, deflated my soul,
being awake all night has taken its toll.
But that's my condition, quite a struggle,
It leaves my writing all in a muddle,
last night I had nightmares, painful you see,
- please leave me alone, I just want to be
by myself all night and all day, too,
my doctor tells me this I will rue,
but this is simply how I want to be,
- damn the lot of them – I want to be ME.

Lightly I Tread

Lightly I tread as on eggshells
for you have a bout of depression
my love for you is undiminished
but I have a good suggestion,
why don't I hug you for comfort
why don't you just take my love
for you are you in your sadness
but you are as gentle as a dove.
I hold your warm hand in your pain
I hold your warm heart under strain:
sleep on my sweet lovely if you can,
all this I want to make plain.
I'm standing by you in these bad moments
for you are the love of my life,
I'll stand by you in your sad moments
we married in health and in strife.
I look at your face and I marvel
at the beauty of humankind,
I look at your body and love you
- can't get you out of my mind.
Depression is here to visit
I'm sticking by you to the last,
for you need love and comfort
for the future and for times past.
My love, I tread lightly as on eggshells
I pray for you as I kneel,
you don't need to talk or say anything
- my support for you, you can steal.

LIKE A FINE PIECE OF CHINA

Like a fine piece of china, my mind's broken now;
it's happened: I know not why nor how.
My mind was priceless, sharp and fast,
now I'm reduced to living in the past.

Like a piece of fine china, it cannot be mended
no matter how I try, no matter how it's tended;
I can cover-up the damage, to make it look neat
as I go to the garden and take to my seat.

I muse and I brood, how it used to be:
I muse and I curse as I sip my tea;
I muse and I blame no one else for the crime
the experts still tell me I'll be better in time.

My mood swings are instant, my thoughts are not strong
I'm impatient today, for days past I long
when I was so hardy, efficient and neat
but now I am scared to go on the street.

The psychiatrist has diagnosed a condition so mean
it's shaken my confidence, it remains to be seen
how I will manage from one day to the next
I look at my booklet and follow the text

On how one should manage one day at a time
I'm not concentrating, why it doesn't even rhyme;
My mind it is broken and I'm sad at the thought
I'm aghast at the symptoms that reduced me to nought.

I fear for my future: I may not be sane,
I'm so focused on problems I don't notice the rain;
the rain is a portent of how things might be,
may God in His mercy have pity on me.

John Ryan

Like a fine piece of china that's broken and past
its best days, I feel that I simply won't last
the pressure that's building on me to survive
- if I go on like this I won't be alive

to all that is happening in the world outside
I mused on this earlier and by then I had cried
at the prospect that is looming before my sad face
- were I a believer I would ask God for grace.

But I am a believer, yet I simply can't pray
to the good Lord in heaven that beside me he'll stay;
I am caught in a cycle that's beyond human thought
I'm a piece of fine china that's reduced to nought.

My appetite's withered, the enjoyment is gone
not like days of old when I sang a song
in my heart with great pleasure, now it's no more
self-respect's missing, I'm just a bore.

My memory's gone, my judgement is weak
I feel that I'm just an undisclosed freak;
my breakdown it came from out of the dark
but I want to be normal, yet I'm way off the mark.

I think of the others who, like me, are sick
yet the public at large may see them as thick:
we need education about all these ills
so the public at large will think without frills.

Don't judge me too harshly because I'm unwell
let my condition be seen as a warning bell
to whoever may listen: if it happened to me
it could happen to you, then you won't be free.

Freedom is all, that's all I can say
Be grateful you are keeping mental illness at bay;
Think kindly of those who are caught in the dark,

Like A Fine Piece of China

who are scared to go out for a walk in the park.

Like a fine piece of china, I am not in one piece,
I am broken quite badly - I want a new lease
of life to the full but I don't think it'll be
think kindly of others, think kindly of ME.

John Ryan

MENTAL BREAKDOWN

Strange experience, a complete breakdown,
like a massive earthquake, in slow motion.
The solidity of mundane, everyday life
brought to an end: the process is complex
and slow. Powerful forces at play, the rocks
which marked out the previous certainties
begin to move, questions forming in the mind:
"What's going on, for Chrissake"? The
previous certainties, solid, stable, begin to
liquefy, the psychological solidities begin to
shift and even move, imperceptibly. No one
has an explanation, I get shifty and no longer
trust myself, much less others. Night-time
sweat and bad dreams compound a now
frightening situation, and I experience a slow,
sizzling panic: now that's scary, day or night.

Professionals make psychiatric seismic checks,
who are these people? "Relax – we're here to
help". An aftershock, the reality of being
sectioned, rumbles to my very core: they're
here to help me be sectioned, I assure myself.
Reassurance in full flow – care in the community.
I answer all questions politely, and that evening
I make my bed, first night in a psychiatric hospital.
Shit – I can't recall where this is, let's christen it
Bedlam, it'll do for now. And these guys want me
to sleep: what, now? In my state? I see straightaway
that these fellow-sufferers are, psychologically speak-
ing,
shell-shocked, sleeping in the open air, as it were.
Yes, before you ask, yes I can spell traumatised.
Desperate for a roll-up, I meander to the smoke-

room, and one poor soul asks for a fag "until later".
Against all my instincts I roll the thinnest fag you've
ever seen. I muse: why is he a "poor soul" – are my
mental processes, and is my very language wanting?
Then, worse than the original quake, I hear a Voice
– again. Don't these professionals know I don't do
sleep, not your normal sleep, and certainly not your
normal sleeping hours? They'll find out . . .

To think it's come to this. "no, mate, I'm voluntary"
- famous first words. My Voice is effing and blinding,
and one guy kicks his chair endlessly. I wish he
wouldn't do that, I mean I really wish he wouldn't do
that. My headache comes back in full regalia.
Courteous to a fault, I tell my Voice to f*** off!
"Do it, do it" it shouts again. I jump to the door and
use the first dirty mug I can find to slake my thirst.
I'm beginning to panic, so I squeeze the teabag end-
lessly, stir the sugar endlessly, round and round,
slowly round and round. Shit, my hands are actually
shaking, and they say it's bedtime? Not in my
community of one it ain't. Another rumble – a doctor
wants to see me, well, I've just arrived so maybe the
teams with their sniffer dogs have bits of paper to
fill-in. Not now, surely. "Describe the problem, your
feelings I mean". The Voice won't let up. My problem
is wrong place, wrong time. Bedlam wasn't invented
for the likes of me. I'm so confused I'm institutionalised
already. I can hear a vicious argument down the corri-
dor.

*   *   *   *

A month later, I'm flourishing in my institutionalisation.
That's a big word, couldn't find a bigger one. I know all
the

John Ryan

dosage and have even learnt a new language: I ask, chirpily,
for my Venlafaxine, Aripiprazole, Simvastatin, Metformin
and good old Aspirin (no, they don't play for Arsenal). My
Voice has, apparently, given up – for now. But I've got a
new problem: afraid to go out. My mind has been dissected,
analysed, reformatted, I'm ready to go home. But I don't
want to cross the street. I shall miss Bedlam. Problem is the
new Me is still the old Me, minus the suicide, minus the
Voice - for now. Question is: is that progress? They don't
know I hear the Voice at night. I want out of here, Voice
or no Voice. These aftershocks unsettle me. I'm still living
in the open, yesterday's orthodoxy is today's nagging doubt.
I feel vulnerable, weak, and cannot get used to the traffic.
Maybe Shakespeare had some wise words about the mind.
Must check it out. I feel I have to re-learn from scratch, I
don't feel optimistic. I feel distinctly gloomy. But I'm alive
and maybe a survivor. Survivors are those who pull through,
are they not? They certainly pulled me from some nasty
rubble. Through the night-hours I ruminate upon my predicament. In one sense I did die: no more bland assumptions.
Not even accepting that today's doubt is tomorrow's New
Certainty.

MENTAL DEATH

Alas, no mechanism
in society to enable
me to mourn
the loss
of my Mind.

Grief has assaulted
me, at the very
moment I expected
Compassion to
visit, and stay.

The shock of sudden
mental death.
The shock. The very
trauma
eats my Soul alive.

Surrounded by fellow-
inmates in the
Psychiatric Wing, not
one expresses a
word of condolence.

I am
all alone
in
my
grief.

MOODS

Sometimes I brood and brood
if I'm in a difficult mood:
I suffer from depression
which inhibits my expression.
Time was when I was at peace
I want my depression to cease.
Not as easy at all as it sounds,
my psyche has to climb the big mounds
of dark voices at night on my bed
- sometimes I wish I were dead.
The voices engage me all night
I end-up in a terrible fight
with the forces of darkness right now:
exhausted, I think I shall die
on my bed for comfort I lie,
with no means of escape I can see,
until the morning I will not be free.
When the daybreak comes at long last
I sip coffee and now break my fast
- if only I could be so free
as to go to a cafe for tea.
I cannot go out on my own:
the result of some seeds that were sown
when I was attacked by a man
who was clearly a beast, not a lamb,
Now I am paying the price
it was chance, like a throw of the dice,
I'm not able to forgive and forget
they tell me I should but I bet
they don't know what it's like to be me
I simply pray the good Lord to be free.

My Muse

Come, my Muse, guide me through
 the midnight hour;
pluck for me a literary flower,
my pen will bleed with passion
I'll no longer have to ration
my words; for thou art close to me
that's really how it should be:
just Thou and me, and me and Thee.
Stay with me, my special Muse,
nothing will I Thee refuse,
with Thee so close my ink will flow
and I may write of pain and woe;
for Thou art my midnight friend
my literary garden I will tend,
with diligence to the very end.

NERVOUS BREAKDOWN

I used to be "normal" but now I'm so weak,
I take time as it comes, I live week by week.
My breakdown it came just out of the blue
I'm sad it is me but I'm glad it's not you.

God's in His heaven, the devil's in hell,
this is my story which I want to tell.
I was abused by a man determined to fight
to achieve his objective: sexual delight.

He achieved what he wanted - he was stronger than
me,
he had his vile pleasure and so now you see
why I suffered a breakdown which lasts to this day;
I suffer intensely - that's all I can say.

But I am amazed at the good folk I've met
who told me they love me and that I shouldn't fret.
But you see, I don't know if I can trust anyone:
I live in the darkness away from the sun.

I really do want to trust humankind,
but my trust has been shattered and so has my mind.
I suffer depression as black as can be;
I suffer paranoia - that is the new me.

My memory's gone, I have blackouts as well,
but it gives me release this story to tell.
It's very good therapy to write down my life,
I wish it were happier instead of this strife.

Think kindly, dear reader, of someone like me
who's sitting and staring while under the tree.
Sitting and staring for hours at an end,
for I look for some comfort from you, my dear friend.

Like A Fine Piece of China

Some people can suffer, and still can endure
the most awful privations - they are saints to be sure.
I'm no saint, nor an angel - I am simply just me,
that's why I do suffer, while under that tree.

My memory's gone, my mind is too weak
to bear all this pain, and so I do seek
release from this cross, release from the pain,
I pray to high heaven that I will stay sane.

I'm angry and bitter, yet forgiving and good;
I'm mixed in my emotions, but I know that I should
forgive all the trauma, the hurt and the pain
- I have to do this if I want to remain sane.

I am scared to go out, I am scared of all men,
as I sit in my room which is now just a den;
this is my prison, as I look for the moon
through a long night of suffering which I hope will end
soon.

My psychiatrist he thinks he can fix my mind,
there is every good chance, as he's gentle and kind;
If I could get back to where I used to be
I would be so happy, for I would be free.

Thank you, kind reader, for hearing my tale,
I'm still feeling sad, because I'm quite frail;
but I feel so much better for telling it through,
May the good Lord in heaven look after you.

NIGHT

The night stretches as far as I can see -
far into the distance I'll still be awake.
Sleep stalks me, even paces the room
with me, but when I grasp her, she
elopes, vaporises in front of my eyes.
Sleep, childlike, likes to play at night,
I put her to bed smartly, and, in foul
mood, I'm resigned to my own
exclusive company. I promise myself
I'll not look at the clock, but I savour
a fleeting glimpse all too often. One
more philosophical fag. Lots to think
about – but hey! we analysed that
last night, and the night before, and
the night before that. The hell with it,
I've got all night, dopey though I am.

The poets and philosophers
gave Sleep a capital letter: such
was their appreciation of the gifts she
showers on some. We've had a stormy
relationship in recent times, since my
paranoia took hold. Sleep takes me
prisoner day-time, sometimes. When
I'm freed, she doesn't even apologise.
I resist always, I detest her, but in
secret I love her, or rather would for
one night's peace.

The demons are out to play, and play
with me. The moon scurries through
the clouds on its epic journey, but I
am left pondering the universe alone.

Like A Fine Piece of China

Paranoia, insomnia, agoraphobia:
all my friends gather for an all-night
feast. Other demons let themselves
in. I put the kettle on and the fun
starts. Sleep refuses to play ball. I'm
too tired to play host. I let them run
riot. They need no encouragement.
In the interests of philosophical dev-
elopement, one more roll-up. One
quick glance – ten past two. Why,
we haven't warmed to the task yet.

The party is a distraction – I want to
be alone. But they crowd me out,
drink my tea and nick my fags. Ex-
pletives fill my conversation, until
Voices kick the door in. Nasty lot,
Voices. Sometimes, in mortal fear,
my hands start trembling. Farewell
the pleasures of quiet meditation.
Come, sleep, get rid of the lot of
them. But no – too much to ask.
And it's not 3 o'clock yet. I notice
Agoraphobia has succumbed to
snoring, but he'll be active all day
tomorrow, so ensuring I'm a
prisoner at home all day. These
demons are having a whale of a
time – and laughing at me, to boot.

Sleep knows full well she's my only
hope, but sniggers at me. Then she
leaves altogether. I know in my
bones she won't be back – not until
the sun is up. Despair whispers sal-
aciously in my ear. That's all I need.
Against advice, I'm having one more

John Ryan

roll-up. Damn the lot of them. One
more tea. By now, I'm in rotten mood.
The Voices are out of control: they're
screaming in my head. The language
is not fit for publication. At 4 o'clock,
there's nowhere else I can go: I'm truly
a prisoner in my bedroom. Scared of
going out at any time, my home is not
my castle at 4 a.m. And I wait for the
first glimmer of day-break. The Light
is one of my trusted friends, but never
hurries, indeed deliberately dawdles.

The Voices drown out any pleasure, but
hey! methinks Sleep has returned. Down
I lie, but no - the one shrill Voice just
won't let up. Now I'm wide awake again.

Another night marked up.

NIGHT WATCH

Again, I'm up at half-past two,
It's snowing hard outside;
I'm wide awake, the Muse is here
And two huge worlds collide.

The world of wake, the world of sleep
Collide this very hour:
But I do want to be awake
To visit my Muse's bower.

I want to have the gift from her
Of eloquence supreme,
I hope that she will see fit now
And notice how I'm keen.

Ye gods, let us commune this hour
When most of mankind sleeps,
I am wide awake just now
The rest are sleeping deep.

Grant me the gift of eloquence
Which I shall tend to well,
My Muse do come and share with me
- A tale that I shall tell.

Obsession

And I loved you so much:
then came my depression,
now I lack expression
adequately to love you
the way I used to . . .
intoxicated with my
problems, I never, ever
lost my obsession for you,
never will . . . deeply in
love I am, still, but deeply
in depression, so weak by
now, trying to be strong
for you. The pain, the
numbness, is worth it just
to share one moment with
you . . .

Oh! ye gods

Oh! ye gods take heed in my hour of need
I am in depression and pain,
I come for assistance and pay my respects
I'm classified as unstable and insane.

Oh! ye gods, I plead, plant a new seed
in my mind so I'll be normal:
then I won't be depressed, or wholly insane
and then I can be quite formal.

Oh! ye gods, I ask, here's a new task:
make me normal and pleasant to be
near my friends and companions and all others too
- normal they all want me to be.

Oh! ye gods, I pray, help me to stay
on the right side of normality all day;
right now I'm locked-up, and fully fed up
my rights may be taken away.

This psychiatric ward is full of some folk
who can't help the way they are,
I want to go home, and be all alone
please don't leave me here with a scar.

Oh! ye gods, I do plead, stay on my side
as others my mind do dissect;
I'll be here for a month – too long it's to be
ye gods choose me among the elect.

Oh! ye gods, I do beg, let me be me
the white-coated folk don't agree:
they say I must alter and be someone else
dammit! Why can't I be just ME ?

John Ryan

Oh! ye gods, I do cry, I don't want to lie
I want to tell the full truth,
I'm stuck in this hell-hole for one full month
my poor mind I ask ye to sooth.

Oh! ye gods, I do say, help me to pray
if that will help me be free:
let me go free, I'm as sane as can be
my wife she is waiting for me.

OPTIMISM

I know you suffer deeply now
but I am here to caress your brow,
I love the times we spend together,
my love is for you, not for another.
Depression is an evil thing
I hope that for you I can bring
some hope, some peace, and ease your pain
- one day I know you'll again be sane.
For I am optimistic now, so
in time I know you won't feel so low,
for you are a fighter, the dark you will fight,
one day soon you'll come to the light;
and when that day comes you'll emerge from that hole
to greet the new dawn – and capture my soul.

Optimistic

Depression I fight
as I wait for the light,
I fight pain and scorn
as I enter the morn,
a brand new day
as on my bed I lay,
I'm a born fighter:
this makes my load lighter,
determined, optimistic,
I'm not pessimistic,
it's going to be a good day,
that's what I have to say.
A day full of promise,
if I am to be honest,
a day full of pride,
heaven knows, I have tried
to be optimistic,
and not pessimistic,
as I gaze at the ceiling
I feel I am healing
slowly, at last . . .

PARANOIA

They say I'm paranoid, I say I'm just normal - but cautious. I'm sure he, or someone like him, can even now, get me. I sit in my home day and night, but am happy in my own company:

I'm happy to be at home
but sometimes I'd like to roam
outside in the wind and the sun
- now that would be such fun;
but now it's all over for me:
they say I'm delusional, you see,
I no longer go out and about
all because of this nasty lout
who assaulted me one fine day,
one day I am sure he will pay.
I had a nervous breakdown -
began acting like a demented clown,
but I'm now on the mend
and so greetings I send
to all fellow-sufferers out there
as I suffer depression in my lair
"keep up the good work" is my
message to you all
remember that you can walk tall,
just like me, you can be on the mend,
Good Luck, from another new friend.

Peace

Today I'm in a very strange mood
I need a hand my pain to sooth,
it's the start of a brand new day
I want to ensure I don't go astray;
so I look to my friends on PsychCentral to ease
my way to hope, and a modicum of peace.
Gather round, friends one and all,
massage my grumpiness, and help me walk tall,
my depression is deep, my pain is intense,
with the help of my friends I may see some sense.

Trauma

"Come" the demons said, "come share with us" on grassy slopes
and re-live times when demons ruled and demons ran amok within
the soul. These times are too traumatic to re-live: spring's gentle
face calls forth a newer start with spurts of sudden sun-shine.
Massage my soul, I yearn – the holding-house of evil spirits for
far too long.

"Come play with me", a demon said, "let's play on grassy slopes
like days of yore". "Begone" I snap, "And come no fur-ther now"
Tormented soul, much weaker from the pain, tired, and sleepy too,
cries out "Begone!" But still the demons come in droves, intent on
victims – even me, even now.

On grassy slopes the memories are etched of former trauma for the
mind: one last gasp "Begone" as a ray of sunlight falls upon my pen
beckoning me outside to charge my brain with spring-time air and rid
myself of demons, sprites and all such forces of the night.

Why make the former times the future times when springtime winds
can blow the soul to future climes and better sleep?

Come, come,
deep Sleep, and read my need for deeper sleep on
grassy slopes
devoid of demons, sprites and such.

No more trauma, no more pain, no more demons out to
play on
slippery slopes. Come to me a slumber deep, come and
ease my
pain - at least until the dream is o'er.

Retreat

I want to retreat from all the pain
I need to be solitary once again,
I need some space to be just me
I go to the kitchen and make some tea.
Now I'm away from all the fray
I'll have peace on my own all of the day,
nothing will distract me from the task in hand
as I attend to my life, on my bed I land.
Some folk may think this is not right
but I'm scared to go out, and have to fight
my demons, I have to face alone
- the result of seed that was earlier sown,
in my room I am more than happy to be
enjoying my company, for that is ME.

SECTIONED

A friend of a friend is "Sectioned"
under the Mental Health Act:
A way of life imposed, what was
No longer is; what is, is born of
Desolate grief. What will be, will
Be for the foreseeable future.

My memories are raw.

Loss of sleep, of appetite, of the
Will to live, on suicide watch.
Being looked-at, gaped-at.

Avoiding eye-to-eye response,
At any cost. So disconcerting.
And society, to top it all, is
So suspicious.

September

September shows a milder side:
her gentle beams of rare sunshine
coax me to my garden retreat:
I lie low.

After great trauma, such mildness
comes as a shock - afraid to upset
Milady lest she turn on me with
a drenching.

The very stones show greater
calm than I. The very stones
reproach me for my timidity.
"Relax" she whispers in the wind.

Nature heals in unexpected ways.
The unexpected sun resonates
with me. September may still
make me whole.

SEXUAL ASSAULT

I'm really scared to go outside
- don't think this is some form of pride
(I wish it were) but sadly not
they tell me that I've lost the plot.
Sexual assault: oh, what a thing!
the thought, it causes bells to ring
within my psyche, deep inside,
some folk maintain that I have lied.
Little do they know how much I've cried
upon my bed when I've been tired.

Today I cannot face the road
outside my house for I am told
by voices deep within my head:
going out I really dread.
The voices shout and scream at me:
to ease the pain I make some tea
for consolation from the pain
I stay inside in sun and rain.
I pray the gods they keep me sane.

I hope that they will hear my sigh,
I hope that I may cease to cry;
each morning, noon and evening die
a tortuous death with no good-bye
to all my friends who love me well
instead I shuffle to my cell
in hope of sleep to hold me fast
from nightmares that all night do last:
tonight's the same as all nights past.

I so much want to walk the street
- that would be such a precious treat;
but I was so assaulted then

it makes me scared to be with men.
I simply do not trust the folk
- if I walk the street I sometimes choke
inside my mind, for I am weak,
exhausted, now escape I seek
It's not a form of pride, but meek
I am, today, and all the week.

The voices shout out "Get this man"
I've done my best, no more I can
endure this life, what's left of it;
that I be safe, and serve no writ
- instead I plead my mind be lit
forgiveness is the sacred bit,
I muse, as on my bed I sit.

Sometimes I think what's best for me
would be found hanging from a tree
- such is the pain, such is the loss
of innocence, as soft as moss.
The voices come again and shout
"Do it! do it!" out aloud:
I'm scared in case the others hear
- I'm scared and closer to a tear.
Right now I am consumed by fear.

I stay inside my house all day
and keep the evil man at bay.
Perhaps he's grinning in my face
his work was done, he left no trace,
but still I can't forgive the fact
(against the scripture's holy tract)
My soul's so full of anger now
my mind recalls the tenet "Thou
shalt forgive the wrong":
It fills my soul just like a song

I cannot do it, all I long
is to hear it whispered on my tongue.

But I am scared, and I am weak,
scared of streets, I'm just a freak
who scowls around the garden now,
I clean the sweat from off my brow
It's here I'm safe from humankind
It's here I cleanse exhausted mind.
I doze upon my table wide
I fantasize that angels side
with me in battle with the depths
maybe they'll help me with my steps
toward sanity, I wish they would
and maybe then I really could
walk the streets like I really should.

Sexual Assault (2)

My psychiatrist and social worker asked me to put in
poetic form the awful sexual assault, as therapy to en-
able me to face the reality of what happened. I have to
say I found this quite traumatic. . .

One September morning
it came without warning,
Thrown against a wall,
unprepared for a fall:
had my trousers pulled down,
my attacker had his pleasure,
this was nothing to treasure,
it went on for ages
against all advice from sages;
indecent, immoral, incredible,
that's what happened that September morn,
I felt the butt of scorn,
a victim so unclean
- this was something I'd never seen,
today I carry the scars,
the trauma still mars
my mind, but oh! the pain,
will I ever again be fully sane?
the gods looked down and remember
what happened that morn in September,
feels like they've deserted me,
now I feel no longer free.
Now I am no longer clean,
the dirtiest I've ever been:
a sexual assault one September morn
now I'm totally forlorn.
Perhaps I shall never recover
sometimes I live it all over

again: that's the result of a sexual assault
but it's not how I ought
to be, I must fight
to get to the light.
Be kind to me in my pain,
for I want to return to be sane.
I cannot write about this well
- a better poet would better tell
this gruesome tale, strange but true,
I want it finished and start anew . . .

SLEEP

Come, deep sleep, deep-cleanse
my soul with rest, for I am tired
of life just now; I need to distance
myself awhile and renew.

You have evaded me lately, I
was so busy: that's my excuse.
It was I who evaded you.
But you always win in the end.

Take hold of my body, take me
gently, help me unwind from
life's affairs, for life without
you is impossible. I marvel at

your ability to hold us to
account so that in the most
unlikely places and circum-
stances we fall for your charms.

Come, Lady of the moon-lit
hours, take me on your journey
to a half-conscious, mysterious
state of peace, common to all

living things. Some folk avoid
you, even fight you, to no avail.
You, milady, always win in the
end. I want to caress you:

envelop me in your embrace,
and all will be peace.

John Ryan

Staring

I stare out of my window in the morning
I do exactly the same at night;
some people say that they love me
-but I'm a pathetic sight.

I'm racked by depression in the morning
kept awake by paranoia at night,
I keep looking from that window by day
having greeted the morning light.

The feeling of numbness is overwhelming
I certainly don't feel all right,
think of me in my discomfort
as I wait for that morning light.

My struggle with depression is so demanding
that I cannot even manage a bite,
my appetite's gone, like much else
I want to give up the fight.

I know this is not a good sign
as out of my window I stare,
I'm alone all day at that window
while no one understands, nor do they care.

On reflection I'm sure that isn't quite true
as many friends on the net will agree,
but depression is nasty in all of its forms
as my friends they all want me to be

healthy, and happy and wise as a sage
I can't measure up to the task,
so I wallow in pain from that window by day
as I drink warm tea from my flask.

Like A Fine Piece of China

If only I could get rid of depression
my life would change utterly overnight:
my friends on the net mean so much to me
I'm going to log on to that site.

I shall meet all of them as they go day by day
I shall greet them and be very kind,
we will stand by each other for that's what it's for
 - THEY will help me to mend my poor mind.

Sunrise

The sun filters through the window,
rays bouncing off the chandelier,
but my soul has a monochrome
existence. That soul is war-weary,
hungry, scars all over.
Is there ever to be a respite?
When will the bugler call a halt?
When will my misty depression lift?
When will the sun nourish my mind?
When will the dew evaporate from
my sodden soul?
Numb is my soul after great pain.
After great pain comes a soothing,
lesser pain. . .
My soul is now immune to pain.
Depression permeates the ego, yet
the early sun impresses me with
its potential. . .
the fire in the crystal chandelier
keeps my mind from existential darkness,
the sun has warmed me sufficiently for
the battles ahead.
My pen is oozing with positive vibes,

Sybil

I want to know everything,
but what if to no avail?
I want to know enough
to survive my melancholy.
The fascination of knowing
all there's to know: would
I swap it all to be free from
melancholia?

Too close to call. Now come
the Muses near to me
this hour of deepest
melancholy. O Sybil, let
me see your cave,
 and wail no more and
do not rave, for here I
wallow in my room, I
need you to my life approve.

Cast me out no more I plead:
instead I want my case appealed.
Darkened cave for darkened deeds,
take me past the rustic reeds,
 where we can play the lyre alone,
my melancholia will by then be gone.

Tell Me Why

Tell me why I'm so depressed
today, I know you're not impressed
with me as I suffer the most awful strain:
I love you, but is my love in vain?
You, too, love me - and not in vain
I'm going through the most awful pain
as depression eats my soul and mind;
it helps that you are to me so kind:
without you I don't know what I would do,
- fortunate indeed as there are few
who really understand my plight,
gives me courage to put up a fight
and enables me to carry on today;
and now upon my bed I'll lay:
reflect on those who wish me well
for I to them have a story to tell
one day, about the power of love,
about you, my dear, my innocent dove;
don't fly away from my abode -
stay here with me as I bear my load
gladly and happily: we'll be together
- just you and me: birds of a feather.

THE DREAM

For I would love to dream
The dream of dreams,
The dream to crown them all;
All my friends would be there
Happy, cheerful, the way
The dream of dreams would
Have it.

Happy to replace the nightmare
All so common: happy to
Replace the half-dreams, not
So happy, cheerful, the way
With half-dreams.

For I would love to dream all
Night and dream again that
All is well with friends who
last the test of time.

THE MANY TIMES

The many times when I did think of life's weird ways,
Upholding stern belief in peoples' better selves -
It's a truth worth holding to. The many times the
Opposite seems true, but we hold a sacred trust to
Bring the fruits of love to bear upon a sceptic
Crowd.

Weird indeed, the many times when good folk snap
The cord that binds us all, and forever disappear.
Who knows, their better selves shine forth for us to
Hold the cord that frays in places, severely so, yet I,
Good and bad, manage to hold on, if barely so at times.

The many times.

THE POEM WITHIN

Deep within the breast
lies a secret thought,
a nugget of fine wisdom
anxious to escape. If
only I could catch the
moment now, and
place it on the page
fresh and struggling to
survive. A fervid mind
struggles to create the
pearl of wisdom for a
moment's gift, to hold
a phrase so accurate
before it's lost
for e'er.

John Ryan

THE PSYCHIATRIC WARD

I remember my days in the psychiatric ward,
I look back without fear or dread. Now I am
Much improved, enjoying life and every bit
Of it. A far cry from those October days. How
Life changes: then, we feared for life itself,
Now we fear losing the zest for life.

Inevitably, autumn is remembrance time, the
Fall from sanity itself. As I then gazed at
The trees I loved every moment, the sheer
Colour and scale of movement as a myriad
Leaves fell and graced the ground. A happy
Interlude.

Those leaves, multi-coloured and of such
Delicacy, now long-forgotten: even in freefall
They offered such delight in those unhappy
Days. I painted them with exquisite care.
My one and only source of delight in an abysmal
situation. Who could compose exquisite poetry
In such conditions?

And yet, the Spirit survived and survives to this hour.
Perhaps my Muse will take pity . . .

The Bully

The bully fine-tunes his craft
in ways subtle and mean;
waiting at life's crossroads
with his cohorts at the ready.
Dark alley for a dark alley mind
- the moon fails to oblige.
Suits him fine, he's in his
element, in rainy mood,
and, like the rain, stubborn,
persistent, repetitious to
tedium. His grunt is generosity
personified. The dripping trees,
seeing all, are forever
struck dumb on the spot.
His eloquence, in snarling
yelps, achieves a chorus
of compliance, while he
complies with the rituals
of respectability. Easy victims,
easy prey, tight-chested,
attempting to evade. The
structures invite, ensure,
 eventual confrontation.
Fear, guilt: a blanket to
cover the mind's confusion
- the weakest link in the
armoury of defence.
Respectability's collusion:
the knotweed choking
the rose.

John Ryan

The City Street

The city street
is all noise and ceaseless
energy: my soul yearns for
the priceless energy of quiet
and peace. A suffering
mind negotiates the city not
at all well: it craves calm, so
alarmed at the decibels
spewn forth, as not to want
to repeat. My mind is
screaming, my body is
restless - blown off course
by the noise and pollution.
If I don't retreat I shall hit
the rocks of raw panic, en-
gulfed by naked fear. I
retrace my steps with quiet
deliberation. Welcome, home.

THE GODS AND MUSES

For I would fain have wished for better times
And yet the gods they smile on me, if only
I could see. Though all alone, I still have Muses
Smiling down on paltry efforts to placate
These gods. The mind is slow and lazy
This early morning hour, but I am happy
in such company. If only I could see the gifts
They grant and respond accordingly . . .

Come, my favourite Muse, and teach me
All those steps which lead to grace and favour
With the gods. Then, these will be better times
Indeed. Come, the light of day, this early morning
Hour: come the sun and warmly shine on creatures
Such as me in my forlorn abandonment.

Sweet Muse, that I may know the secret ways
To curry favour with the gods. Come and spread
Thy favours lavishly on me and I shall give my very all
In recompense.

Come, sweet Muse: be kind to me
and we will please the gods this very hour.
Sweet verses we will pen and tell of all the goodly hours
Spent deep in valleys of Arcadia.

John Ryan

The Long, Long Road

I went down the long, long road
and by my side you were in sombre mood
We stopped, and looked in each other's soul
Your face showed that life had taken its toll,
but I wanted you on this path with me
- thou with me and me with thee.
I know you suffered from depression,
me? I wanted to relieve you from oppression
if only for the duration of this walk
-so stay with me and we can talk.
In your eyes I see the faintest smile:
come on, let's walk another mile
and then we can rest and see those eyes
of yours properly; there will be no more lies
from me, for when I tell you, forsooth,
that I love you, it is nothing but the truth.
I see the first teardrop, but now: no more tears
- hold me, and I will relieve your fears
in one warm hug, you will see my mind
and my tears, too, for my heart is kind
to you, and that beautiful face now lined
with life's furrows, I hope you don't mind
if we sit here; we have all day, love isn't timed
for only you exist on this long, long road
and now you are in happier mode.

THE MORNING AFTER

The nights are the worst of it:
depression sets in, and I count
the hours, sometimes the
minutes. I'm up before the first
bird in the morning, exhausted.

A breakdown alters everything
and apparently everyone, or so
I think. It's certainly altered me.
No more refreshing Shakespeare's
sleep, instead the deep, deep
depths of night despair. Alone
I ruminate, meditate, philosophise,
and count the cigarette butts -
each a testament to hours of
introspection.

I'm moody, tired now, tired of
life, for sure, moody such that
my way with words has evap-
orated, temporarily. The phone
rings, and I try to sound chirpy,
but nature betrays me once
again. Let nature do me a favour
and give me sleep while the
world rush-hour is underway.
The morning after sees me at
my most vulnerable. You
should see me: I look anything
but venerable.

Stoically, I know tonight will
see the same pattern, and the

night after, for this is the new
Me. Even the postman brings
sober, boring news: the sun,
summery-like, is alone in
smiling at everyone. I trust
no one and smiling is, for me,
an ancient craft long since
lost through sheer neglect.
Even an early-morning shower
will not lift the cloud of
depression.

To think of all I've lost, and
at what cost . . .
To think of what I've gained:
something approaching a
deeper insight into what
makes me tick. As long as I
don't mention the morning
after. Exhausted, I'm too
tired to cover-up, so much
so I don't even want to dress
for that rush-hour. Don't be
fooled, I lie: I don't do rush-
hours anymore.

Instead, I am alone and
deliriously happy at the
prospect, as long as you call
me once the morning fog
has lifted. Depression
weighs me down, I cannot
move, so it's tablet-time,
dosing myself while rush-
hour participants clamber
to their factories to make
me more. I've got God's

calling card, but cannot
summon the strength to
smile at Him.

My psychiatrist has all the
answers, all I have are all
the questions: "why ME"?
I'm not impressed with all
the psycho-babble. I'm too
numb, it's over my head this
morning. Tell me in the
afternoon. If only I could
break out of this pit. Why
then I would be fit to join
the rush-hour. But no, thank
you: I want to be alone. It's
the morning after.

The Muse

Sitting in my small garden of delights,
seems the Muse has left me temporarily
but I have my many friends at PsychCentral
to remember, to console me in my
loneliness, for they are kind, good folk,
and that thought is with me, sustains me
in my social isolation.

The Prescription

I walk with my stick in hand
to collect my prescription;
the mist encloses round,
keeping the mood solemn.

No more birds for company
- they've flown south for winter,
even the squirrels seem to have
abandoned these parts.

My progress is slow, deliberate:
this official paper equates to an
assurance of medication, to keep me
on a level mental state.

My future assured, for now at least,
my past signed-off, my present
reflected in the weather, changeable.

THE RAIN

The rain is pelting on the window hard,
And I can hear the wind throughout the house;
An hour ago, the sun it brightly shone
- All so quiet, one could hear a mouse.

The change it came so suddenly,
The wind came up so quiet,
The dazzling sun then disappeared
And lo! We lost the light.

It makes me think of life's strange ways,
The way things come to pass,
And I am here so all alone
- The raindrops fall en masse.

They press against the window pane,
And dance in rivers down:
My former visage happy, bright,
Is replaced now with a frown.

And yet, as I do pen these words,
The blue sky distant shows;
The garden's got a sprinkling
- So did my favourite rose.

Sunshine and showers: that's what they said,
This time they got it right;
This episode has now gone past,
My room is full of light.

THE WILD MOORS

Too many times I wandered
the wild moors
alone,
too many times I tempted
the weather
and survived dry;
too many times I heard Voices
and panicked,
wind in my face,
eating my bald head,
now I am content - at least for now.

Too many times I struggled
uphill,
too many times I was scared
of my Voice,
now I am in control
while the rain lashes my soul,
now I am content – at least this hour.

Too many times I gave way
to the Voice,
too many times I didn't understand,
now I am master of the Voice
while the clouds gather
ominously,
now I am content – at least this trek.

Too many times I heard
the souls who got lost here,
too many times souls got lost
in the mist,
too many times a haunting Voice

John Ryan

whispered,
but I am content – at least on this rest.

Too many times I've trekked
this slushy path,
too many times I've watched
as it came to dusk,
the curlew distant far,
not many times a screaming Voice was
conquered,
but I am content: now I am in control.

I am content on the wild moor
as the clouds disperse once more,
these days I talk to my Voice
as one
not like the days of yore.
Now I am content:
dark on the moor
but bright in my soul.

With the wind on my back
and a song on my lips
I come off the wild moor
at last;
I have faced down my Voice
with the wind as a friend
now I am content:
it's passed.

The Wind

The wind blows cold on my mind
but I don't care - it's a kind wind,
 mellow and gentle, joined by the
soft rain already signed by the
forecast.
The wind blows cold on my soul,
but I don't care - it's a strong soul
just now, abundantly sprinkled by
the rain.
The wind blows cold on my face
but I don't care - it's a rugged face
through years of pain, accustomed
to wind and rain.
The wind blows cold on my conscience
but I don't care - it's a clean, sober
conscience knarled by years of
prudent, if sometimes crafty, decisions.
The wind is a metaphor for the journey
of my soul: now strong, now weak,
sometimes not moving for days on end;
othertimes enduring a storm from which
there is no escape. The wind is my friend.
When in great pain, the wind on my back
is a helping hand. After great pain, the wind
on my face welcomes me home.

John Ryan

The Wind Blows Gentle

The wind blows gentle on my face,
it's summer time, the wind blows
warm on my face, reflecting the
warmth and gentle disposition in
my soul. Today's a warm and gentle
day. My roses in my garden of delights
give off a warm and gentle scent . . .
if only I could hold on to this,

Like A Fine Piece of China

To All My Friends

The deep, deep pit is black and dark,
my depression has definitely left its mark;
now I'm not writing anymore
I've become one lazy, sad, bad bore.

My reversal is sadly out of my control,
I'm in the darkest depression inside my soul:
I need all the friends I've got on the net
so I don't fall deeper, and no longer fret.

Rapid mood swings are now part of me,
one day up, one day down, it's like that you see,
when I'd down I'm depressed like you'd not understand:
I know depression like the back of my hand.

There's that feeling of numbness, a weight so heavy
I can't keep control, my hands are not steady:
I look to my friends on this site for peace:
think kindly of me as a new life I lease.

Too Often

Too often I spread my wings to fly
above the clouds; too often my
ambition was thwarted: I fell
to earth with a thump.

Too often I tried to leave my house,
to break my agoraphobia: too often
I turned back in fear of everyone.

Too often I tried to stop my mental
pain, to stave off depression:
vaulted ambition proved my undoing.

Too often I forced myself to sleep
all through the long night: too often
I greeted the first sunbeams, exhausted.

Too often I had ambitions for a great
poem; too often I waxed lyrical with the
Muse: too often I got writers' block.

Too often I tried to be a new "me"; I
tried so very hard; too often I had to
modify my ambition, for I too often
had to settle, negotiate with the old "me".

Too often the old "me" defended its
territory, in defiance of the upstart;
too few times I've learned to love the old "me".

VOICES

The voices seldom come these days
but when they do we speak on equal terms -
not like former times. The former times
are best forgot and yet, and yet it seems to
me: recalling them is therapy indeed. The
hell they meant to me is now subdued, for
I've learnt to negotiate a truce between my
rational self and the side that would drive a
mind insane.

Rose-tinted glasses are no option for this
poet, alas. The truth is stated as it is, devoid
of ornament. A hounding voice is one from
hell – or so it was when fear, confusion,
even panic reigned supreme. Four long years
it took to gain a portion of my mind back for
myself.

Reflecting now, amazement sets the setting
for a new, bright winter's day when otherwise
all hell would greet my slumber's end. Ye
gods, that I may sober stay and not to panic
and its pain give way. These voices, now
subdued, we now negotiate the whys and
wherefores of our times – together and
apart. A shouting voice still shocks, but now
there is resemblance of a truce, a partial
pact that gives control to me, such that I can
greet my voice and have civil conversation.

The days – and nights – of sweaty fear are
o'er and now I see the voices for what they
are. Begone the times of mortal fear,
welcome times of goodness to hold dear

hoping that a wholeness deep inside
is very near.

VOICES (2)

The Voices come to me at last:
and I'm shaken to the core
and shocked, overwhelmed,
now I don't know what's in store.

Benevolent or otherwise, who's
to say? A Voice screaming at me
- far from benevolent – telling
me to "Do it! Do it" don't you see?

They told me to acknowledge and
negotiate – keep the Voice at bay;
now I'm in such a state,
what am I to say?

I shall keep calm and talk, but
not show the shock and the fright;
these are very good tactics
I'll take the Voice on and fight

to show who's in control,
to show I am not beat;
now I am famished and shaking
- I don't pretend as I seat

myself down on my bed and
let the Voice ramble away;
I'm in control of my life:
it will not lead me astray.

and so I answer back for now
"Do it! Do it" it shouts,
as I am getting even more scared
- my mind is full of the louts

who abused me in those far-off
days, now my mouth is so dry;
I think of the future, not the past
and now I am starting to cry.

I sob for a while and then I stop
while I control my emotions;
the Voice is still shouting away
as I attend to my devotions.

Eventually the Voice goes away
as I get up and I kneel down and pray
that the gods will keep me in peace
and be sanguine for the rest of the day.

Voices are frightening and scary
if we don't know what they are;
but now my Voice has departed
forever, I hope, and far.

Winter in My Mind

It's June outside, but it's winter in my heart
and I was hoping to make a fresh start
but now the heat is sizzling hot
yet heat in my soul? I think not.
Not at least for now, for I am deep depressed
- now I'm sitting and despairing, not impressed.
No heat in this room, for it's winter in my mind,
no sun percolating through, my mood is not kind
this hour, I'm in abject desolation;
for this mind, there is no consolation.
O come, console me in this freezing hour,
I'm deep submerged in snow inside my ivory tower.
This is where I live, for I am scared to leave,
this is where I want to die, for I believe
it is too dangerous to venture forth outside
- too busy with my thoughts which I've applied
diligently, which cause me to remain within
and my excuses are seemingly wearing thin,
for people ask me to come and see the sun
"Come", they say, "come and have some fun
with us"; from me, a deafening silence, why?
because I'm ill with negativity, pity me,
"Come and get some sun", they plea
while I struggle and lie on my bed
- to go outside I'm scared, something that I dread.
Folks don't understand, they think I'm somewhat mad
I plead for understanding, for I'm sad, not bad.

Words

Sometimes I think that I think too much,
sometimes I think that I talk too much
to my mind, saturated with words,
not valued. After great pain, words are
jewels, greatly sought after, for they are
few and meaningful . . .
sometimes I think that the groans of
human pain can be eloquent - testament
to simplicity, cutting to the quick, without
elaboration, or the need for such. Pain
yields reduction. Reduction may lead to
wisdom. Words are few at the top
of the mountain of human pain – but
entirely memorable . . .
my wordy mind is capable of endless
 words: severely limited in words that
are meaningful. It may all be said in
one scream, such is the pain: never
was a mind so eloquent as then. It
is understood in every tongue . . .
sometimes I think that I should stop
and scream . . .
ye gods,
that I may know this wordless wisdom in my
wordy mind . . .

WRITING FOR THE MUSES

If I could write the kind of verse
The Muses like to read, the world
Would be a different place indeed.

But its a gift: my Muse dispenses
Such favours cautiously.

The musty stench of Hades' darkened halls
Is all that's left to us to ponder, sometimes,
When the Muses flee and treat us with
Disdain.

But back they come, and we transfer
To sunny uplands, bathed in the glow
Of Love itself.

Now that's a treasure to delight
A sodden soul like mine, this hoary hour,
Writing for the Muses.

John Ryan

YOUR DEPRESSION

My dear, dear friend,
I know the hell you're in,
the black hole
unfathomable,
that weight upon
your tired, tired mind.
Times were, I too
couldn't summon the
strength to climb
the greasy pole to
give me light of day.
I am here to reach
your fingertips
so light may caress
your care-worn brow.
Reach out to me, my
dear, dear friend, take
my worn hand
and heave
one more time.
I love you, we are
inseparable
from now on,
for I love you as you are
- not for what you were
before depression
stormed your soul.
You don't need words
for me, just your hand.
I want to hug you
in your blackest hour
so that, hand outstretched,
you may once more

Like A Fine Piece of China

stand tall
in morning's light,
and smile
- as only you can smile.

Lightning Source UK Ltd.
Milton Keynes UK
16 January 2011
165818UK00001B/12/P